Super Strength Super Fast; Run Faster Jump Higher

Super Strength Super Fast; Run Faster Jump Higher

Eight-Week Exercise Guides
for Sprinting, Jumping, and
Developing Super Strength
through Explosive Weightlifting

Christopher D. McCrane

VANTAGE PRESS
New York

The opinions and instructions expressed herein are solely those of the author. Each individual should seek the advice of his or her own physician before starting any new exercise program.

FIRST EDITION

Super Strength Super Fast was originally published in 1993. *Run Faster Jump Higher* was originally published in 1991. Each was published separately. They are now combined to form the updated 2006 version.

Published by Vantage Press, Inc.
419 Park Ave. South, New York, NY 10016

Manufactured in the United States of America
ISBN: 0-533-15328-X

Library of Congress Catalog Card No.: 2005907435

0 9 8 7 6 5 4 3 2 1

To my parents who pushed me into all sports at an early age. To my older brothers, whose playing of sports allowed me the opportunity to try and break their personal records. To my younger brother, who easily sketched all the art with his incredible artistic ability. To my wife, whose extreme care, love, and patience, allowed me to write this book along with her assistance in typing the many manuscripts. To my uncle, who showed me how to lift weights at the age of twelve, and to the rest of my family who encouraged me to push myself.

Contents

About the Author

Christopher D. McCrane is a former U.S. National and Olympic-qualified bobsledder. While training at Lake Placid, New York, he obtained incredible knowledge from the European and Soviet Union coaches on explosive training techniques used in Olympic-style weightlifting. Olympic-style weightlifters lift enormous amounts of weight with *explosive* speed. Now it is possible to use these kinds of training techniques to develop explosive strength for bodybuilders, powerlifters, and athletes of all sports. The author has over twenty years of weightlifting experience and it has taken him several years to perfect his training regimen. Now you can have these incredible strength gains in *__weeks instead of years!__*

Why I Feel My Books Are Better Than All Others!!!!

1. I incorporate the laws of physics, force = mass times acceleration. (The faster something moves, the more force behind it.)
2. Fast-twitch fibers are the largest, strongest, and fastest fibers. They burn out in the first 5 seconds; they must be exercised within 5 seconds or less. (The fastest exercises incorporate these fibers only!)
3. Plyometric jumps from a height create the fastest reaction times out of all plyometric exercise. (A 200 pound man jumping down from a 6 foot height lands with 50,000 pounds of force! Can you squat 50,000 pounds?)
4. Sprinting downhill creates a longer stride length and a faster turnover rate.
5. Only perform the fastest exercises that create the fastest reactions in the fast twitch fibers. Any exercise that makes your muscles react slower will not make you reach your absolute potential.
6. You must train at 100% on each exercise, and only 3 times a week.
7. Plyometric jumps over boxes or hurdles are not fast enough, and you will never get 100% out of the exercise.
8. Running with a parachute is not one of the fastest exercises; your muscles will react slowly after this training. You will be stronger, with more endurance, but not faster.

9. Running with ankle-weights, weight-vests, and weight-sleds or bungy cords are all resistance exercises that will make you slow.
10. Running up hill is too slow. It shortens your stride and shortens the muscle length.

Conclusion:
> Jogging will make you a better jogger
> Jumping will make you a better jumper
> Sprinting will make you a better sprinter

Muscles have memory, if all they know is fast twitch, then that is what they will do when it is time to do it! They can't give you what they haven't already done!

The doctors and coaches pushing training equipment are probably sponsored by the companies that make them.

If pro-athletes didn't drink Gatorade, would they still be great athletes?

I'm not pushing products because you don't need them to train! **Train smarter, not harder, is the key!!! This comes from experience, not from a doctor!!**

Caution!

This is an advanced weight-training program for the experienced athlete who has trained with weights for at least one year. The athlete beginning this exercise program must train under the strict supervision of a coach, qualified weight-lifting instructor, or partner. Training without a partner may lead to injury and end results may not be as great.

Introduction

This is an eight-week explosive weight-training program designed specifically to give you incredible strength gains! This workout can be used with the bench press, military press, squats, and dead lifts. It has also been used on isolation exercises (i.e., biceps, curls, and triceps extensions) with equally incredible strength gains! Do not be surprised if you gain up to 45 pounds or more on each of the three workouts. Some athletes have actually increased 50 pounds on leg squats after just 2 weeks!

My personal best in the bench press was 280 pounds at a bodyweight of 155 pounds but after only eight weeks it was 400 pounds. One year later I decided to try this eight-week work-out again. My maximum bench press was 425 pounds at a bodyweight of 180 pounds. After completing the eight-week program, I was able to bench press 505 pounds once, and 315 pounds for nineteen repetitions! Incredible results were gained each time.

Regardless of how you have trained before, if you are bench pressing 300 pounds you will be bench pressing around 400 pounds or more using this program. If you are bench pressing 700 pounds you will be bench pressing around 800 pounds or more after eight weeks.

This program must be done in the exact order in which it is outlined. If workout days are missed for any reason, you should start over. Completing this workout for more than eight weeks has not been attempted and results are not available.

It is advised to complete this eight-week workout and then proceed with another (to maintain your strength) for at least one month before repeating this program. Always train with a partner, get plenty of rest, and ***GO FOR IT!***

Super Strength Super Fast;
Run Faster Jump Higher

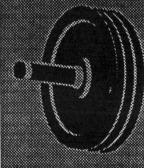
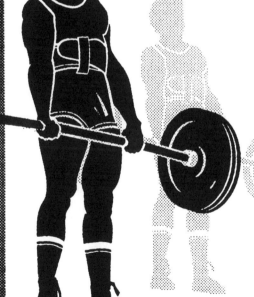

Super
STRENGTH

Super
FAST

An 8-Week
Guide For
Developing
Explosive
Strength

Through
Explosive
Weight-Training

by
Christopher D. McCrane

Absolute Strength vs. Explosive Strength

There are two types of strengths: **absolute strength** and **explosive strength.**

Bulldozers and elephants are both extremely powerful for pushing and pulling, but they move very, very slowly. This is absolute strength. Explosive strength would be the exact opposite. We are talking about thin, muscular, and extremely quick and explosive, like a gymnast, cheetah, or a volleyball player jumping explosively upward in order to spike the ball over the net.

Explosive strength is the creation of a tremendous amount of power in a very short period of time. The faster, farther, or higher you can do something, the more explosive you are. In what sport would anyone need to have absolute strength or brute strength?

Unfortunately, football players think this kind of strength is the best for their sport, even when the explosive players generally make the great plays. Most football players continue to develop absolute strength instead of explosive strength in their weight-training programs. If a 280-pound football player had an absolute strength squat of 500 pounds and his 40-yard dash time was only 5.0 seconds (which is a slow time), I would work more on his explosive strength, making him quicker, and get his 40-yard dash time down to 4.5 seconds or so.

All football players would be much more effective at blocking and tackling if they forgot about the slow, heavy squat routines used a much lighter weight, and did explosive squats. Then, if their squat was 500 pounds explosively, at least they would be faster sprinters than they were before.

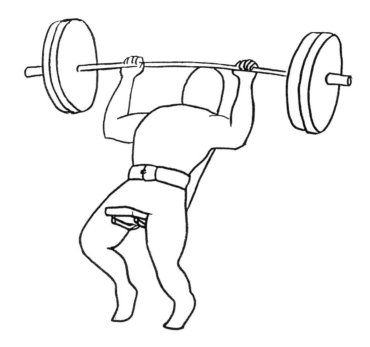

Furthermore, when during any football game have you seen one player squat another player? Football is an explosive sport and explosive weight-training should be the **only** type of weight-training.

Force = Mass x Acceleration

Newton's second Law of Physics, **F = M x A,** states that if the Mass (**M**) is a constant during your "lift" then your Acceleration (**A**) must be increased in order to generate more Force (**F**). This means that you must lift "faster" in order to generate more force. If you are bench-pressing 200 pounds (M), this does not change during the movement. If it takes you one second to perform one repetition, then you will generate 200 pounds of force (F).

$$F = M \times A$$
$$F = 200 \text{ lbs. x 1 second}$$
$$F = 200 \text{ lbs.}$$

If it takes you a "half-second" to perform one repetition, then you are generating 400 pounds of Force (F) just by generating twice the speed. This is when the Olympic style of weight-lifting comes to mind.

The Olympic-style weight-lifter is the perfect example of what explosive weight-training can do for strength. These athletes lift enormous weights with incredible speed but their style of weight-lifting is very difficult and takes a long time to perfect. So, can we apply an explosive weight-training technique to our regular weight-training program in order to create explosive power in specific muscle groups? Absolutely!

The following program can be used for the bench press, squats, dead lifts, military press, and all other exercises. You can become incredibly strong in a very short period of time—***weeks instead of years.***

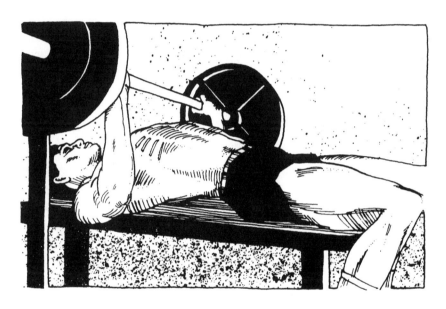

Explode into super strength!

Part 1
Weeks 1 & 2

Before beginning, you must establish your maximum lift or press—that is, the most you can lift or press for one repetition, without the help of a spotter. This weight is equal to 100%. Then you need to determine 60%, 65%, and 70% of this maximum weight. These weights can be exact, or within five pounds less than the exact but never more than the exact. If your maximum is 300 pounds, then 60% of 300 pounds is 180 pounds, 65% is 195 pounds and 70% is 210 pounds.

Perform these repetitions, 5 reps in 5 seconds, *as fast as possible*, with one-minute rest periods between sets. The weights that you will be using and the speed at which you will be lifting them will make this exercise program seem very easy, but since you have never done an explosive lifting routine like this before, you do not know how it should feel. You should complete the two-week routine and then find your "new max." Each repetition should be performed through only three-quarters of full extension of the exercise.

Full extension is not necessary and three-quarters range of motion is a lot faster.

Week 1

Monday	60% of max	5 sets x 5 reps in each set
Wednesday	65% of max	5 sets x 5 reps in each set
Friday	70% of max	5 sets x 5 reps in each set

Week 2

Monday	60% of max	5 sets x 5 reps in each set
Wednesday	65% of max	6 sets x 5 reps in each set
Friday	70% of max	5 sets x 5 reps in each set

The Monday following the Week 2 workout, establish your new maximum lift or press at one repetition. It does not matter if your "new max" is now five pounds or fifty pounds heavier, you are now stronger than you were two weeks ago. This is your goal throughout each of these three workouts.

Part 2
Weeks 3–6

Before beginning Part 2, you should have established your new maximum lift or press for one repetition without the help of a spotter. Using this "new max," you must figure out the proper weights for the following repetitions, but you must follow these easy guidelines.

There will always be a 20-pound weight difference between "even"-numbered repetitions, and a ten-pound weight difference between successive repetitions. The following is an example. If your "new max" is equal to 300 pounds then your weights should be as follows. They must be performed in this order, with a one-minute rest period between sets.

The repetitions are performed *as fast as possible* using a three-quarter range of motion.

> 8 repetitions using 220 lbs.
> 6 repetitions using 240 lbs.
> 5 repetitions using 250 lbs.
> 4 repetitions using 260 lbs.
> 3 repetitions using 270 lbs.
> 2 repetitions using 280 lbs.
> 1 repetition using 300 lbs.

If your "new max" is equal to 250 pounds then your weights should be as follows:

> 8 repetitions using 170 lbs.
> 6 repetitions using 190 lbs.
> 5 repetitions using 200 lbs.
> 4 repetitions using 210 lbs.
> 3 repetitions using 220 lbs.
> 2 repetitions using 230 lbs.
> 1 repetition using 250 lbs.

"If your "new max" is equal to 400 pounds then your weights would be as follows:

8 repetitions using 320 lbs.
6 repetitions using 340 lbs.
5 repetitions using 350 lbs.
4 repetitions using 360 lbs.
3 repetitions using 370 lbs.
2 repetitions using 380 lbs.
1 repetition using 400 lbs.

Use this routine for four weeks, every other day, such as Monday-Wednesday-Friday or Tuesday-Thursday-Saturday. Using same weights for two successive workouts. If, after the second workout, some of the weights were easily completed, or you got the feeling that you might have added one more repetition at that weight, then, on the next workout day, add ten pounds to all the weights that were easily completed. Do not use the same weight for different repetitions. Always add ten pounds in order to make them different. If you are not able to add ten pounds on any weights, continue on to the next workout day until you can add ten pounds to some or all of the weights.

You should be able to add ten pounds to all weights on every third workout. After this four-week workout is completed, you should have added forty pounds to all the weight classes. If your starting maximum weight at one repetition was 300 pounds, then your ending weights should look like the following example:

8 repetitions using 260 lbs.
6 repetitions using 280 lbs.
5 repetitions using 290 lbs.
4 repetitions using 300 lbs.
3 repetitions using 310 lbs.
2 repetitions using 320 lbs.
1 repetition using 340 lbs.

Next again find your "new max" at one repetition. As you know, this is equal to 100%. Then determine 60%, 65%, and 70% of this "new max" and begin your next workout using these new weights.

Part 3
Weeks 7 & 8

You have just found your "new max" again and may now begin your next workout. This is a two-week workout that is exactly the same as the first two-week workout. You can repeat this workout because the four-week workout in between used very heavy weights which could not be performed as explosively as the lighter weights. Thus, there *will* be an improvement again at the end of this two-week workout.

Once again, the repetitions are performed **as fast as possible** with a one-minute rest between sets, using a three-quarters range of motion.

Week 7

Monday	60% of new max	5 sets of 5 reps in each set
Wednesday	65% of new max	5 sets of 5 reps in each set
Friday	70% of new max	5 sets of 5 reps in each set

Week 8

Monday	60% of new max	5 sets of 5 reps in each set
Wednesday	65% of new max	5 sets of 5 reps in each set
Friday	70% of new max	5 sets of 5 reps in each set

Next again find your "new max." Your last "new max" could be 100 pounds or more than your beginning max during Week 1. This routine could be continued for another six weeks, and then another, but I suggest that you begin a completely different program for one month before returning to this workout program.

Conclusion

Explosive weight-training can give you a great deal of extra strength in a very short period of time. This type of explosive weight-training is not being used at the professional or collegiate levels, and definitely not at the high school or junior high school levels. Russian athletes have been using this type of explosive weight-training for decades and it is only now available to the United States through this manual.

The sooner the athlete begins this type of weight-training, the sooner he or she will reach higher levels of competition. Using this type of training, it is likely that in the years to come, champions will be younger than ever. World records will be shattered by younger athletes, and older athletes will be able to compete longer.

Be the FIRST athlete, team, or coach to begin this program. ***Don't be the last*** or you will be left far, far behind those who do use this program.

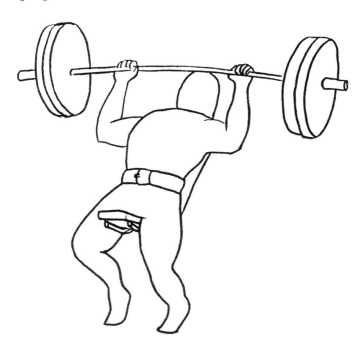

THE BIG FISH
ALWAYS EAT
THE LITTLE FISH!

MAX	1 rep	2 rep	3 rep	4 rep	5 rep	6 rep	7 rep	8 rep

MAX	1 rep	2 rep	3 rep	4 rep	5 rep	6 rep	7 rep	8 rep

MAX	1 rep	2 rep	3 rep	4 rep	5 rep	6 rep	7 rep	8 rep

MAX	1 rep	2 rep	3 rep	4 rep	5 rep	6 rep	7 rep	8 rep

MAX	1 rep	2 rep	3 rep	4 rep	5 rep	6 rep	7 rep	8 rep

MAX	1 rep	2 rep	3 rep	4 rep	5 rep	6 rep	7 rep	8 rep

MAX	1 rep	2 rep	3 rep	4 rep	5 rep	6 rep	7 rep	8 rep

MAX	1 rep	2 rep	3 rep	4 rep	5 rep	6 rep	7 rep	8 rep

MAX	1 rep	2 rep	3 rep	4 rep	5 rep	6 rep	7 rep	8 rep

MAX	1 rep	2 rep	3 rep	4 rep	5 rep	6 rep	7 rep	8 rep

MAX	1 rep	2 rep	3 rep	4 rep	5 rep	6 rep	7 rep	8 rep

MAX	1 rep	2 rep	3 rep	4 rep	5 rep	6 rep	7 rep	8 rep

MAX	1 rep	2 rep	3 rep	4 rep	5 rep	6 rep	7 rep	8 rep

MAX	1 rep	2 rep	3 rep	4 rep	5 rep	6 rep	7 rep	8 rep

MAX	1 rep	2 rep	3 rep	4 rep	5 rep	6 rep	7 rep	8 rep

MAX	1 rep	2 rep	3 rep	4 rep	5 rep	6 rep	7 rep	8 rep

RUN FASTER

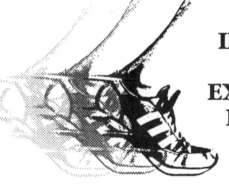

**IMPROVE
YOUR
EXPLOSIVE
POWER:**

*An Eight Week Exercise Guide For
Sprinting And Jumping*

JUMP
HIGHER

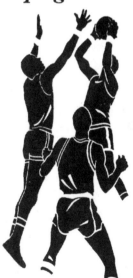

By Christopher D. McCrane

Caution

Consult a physician before beginning any exercise program. Explosive training techniques can and may elevate the heart rate very quickly! Never train alone, and always train under the supervision of a sports coach or athletic trainer for maximum results.

The following exercises must be done exactly as outlined and in order only! The vertical leap can be increased 4 inches or more in just the first week, and 12 inches or more in 8 weeks. Don't be surprised if you get at least a half-second or more faster. Good luck, train smart, and get plenty of rest!

Introduction

All sports require some sort of explosive power whether it's upper body, lower body, running, jumping, or throwing. Swimmers explode off the starting blocks, diving out over the water as far as possible. If a swimmer was able to dive out over the water, beyond half the length of the pool, he/she would most likely win every race. If a swimmer was able to dive out one or two feet farther than all the other swimmers, then he/she would have a distinct advantage.

Divers use explosive power when springing off diving boards. Achieving greater heights in their jumps allows them to have more time to concentrate on re-entry, after performing their flips and spins. All gymnasts, sprinters, hurdlers, javelin throwers, ice dancers, speed skaters, snow skiers, and all track and field athletes use explosive power at sometime during their events. Football, baseball, basketball, and tennis players use explosive power their entire games. The player who can run faster or jump higher usually has a distinct advantage over all other players. Olympic-style weightlifters use explosive power in order to lift enormous weights very quickly. They are said to be the most explosive athletes in the world.

It's quite obvious that all of the greatest athletes in the world, no matter what sport, have either fantastic speed or a fantastic jumping ability. A basic understanding of how the muscles work, and then performing exercises that overload the actions of the muscles, can make an average athlete great and a great athlete an Olympic champion, or high-paid pro. Imagine what a pro basketball player could do if they did some specific running and jumping exercises, and added twelve inches to their vertical leap!

The following exercises are a collection put together after many years of long, hard training. I participated in many sports throughout my childhood, high school, and college. I've also been an avid weightlifter and body builder for almost twenty years. I spent six months training with track coaches, and then spent three months in Lake Placid, New York, at the Winter Olympic Bobsled Training Center.

All of the following exercises were collected during many years of locker room talk, coaching techniques, trial and error, common sense, and articles that were available to the general public in many sports magazines. I performed each exercise in random order, over many months, and at times in much pain. This manual was written based on what worked best for me and should be followed exactly until the entire workout is completed. Then, and only then, should the individual adjust the workout for their own personal development.

There are many books on the subject of running faster and jumping higher. I don't claim to be a doctor of sports medicine, or a graduate of any specialty involving the mechanics of running and jumping. I have not, in any way, plagiarized any book or article on the subject, and any similarity to another book or article is mere coincidence.

Explosive Power

What is explosive power? Explosive power is your muscles' ability to generate or absorb as much energy as possible, and then to release it as fast as possible. When running and jumping, the legs absorb the force generated by this action. The force is then released in the direction needed to propel you either forward or upward, acting exactly like a giant spring.

Plyometrics is the term used to describe this action. Your legs can be considered giant springs that absorb energy, or become coiled. They then spring back, or become uncoiled, in the direction you need. There are many plyometric exercises I have come across that can greatly improve your explosive power and speed in certain movements. You must first develop a strength base before attempting any of these exercises, to prevent any possible injuries.

How do we measure explosive power? We can measure explosive power by measuring our vertical leap. The higher we can jump, the more explosive we are. Short distance running is also a good way to measure explosive power. The faster we can run the more explosive we are. But, I prefer to measure true explosive power by being timed in the 40-yard dash or less. I was timed in a standing start at 4.22 seconds in the 40-yard dash, but my 100 meter time is relatively slow, at 11 seconds or so.

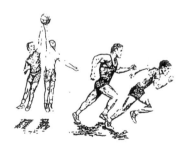

Common Sense Behind the Theory of Explosive Power

Let me try to explain again, in a different way, what explosive power is, and how it works. Let's start with Newton's 2nd Law of Physics.

$$F = M \times A \quad \text{FORCE} = \text{MASS} \times \text{ACCELERATION}$$

When you are jumping, your Mass (M), or body weight, stays unchanged during this action. Therefore, in order to achieve more Force, you must increase your Acceleration. Someone weighing 180 pounds (M), who wants to double (2x) his Force, needs, needs to double his acceleration.

When you double your Acceleration, you are cutting the time it takes in half. An example of this would be running an 8-minute mile and then running a 4-minute mile. Running twice as fast takes half the time.

Let's apply this to jumping. If you were going to try to dunk a basketball, you would have to run toward the basket at full speed, and then convert forward force into upward force. An explosion takes place in your legs, and you are propelled upward. This conversion, let's say, takes exactly one second to complete. Your legs have to absorb the shock of going forward by bending, an eccentric contraction, then your legs have to overcome this force, and covert it into a concentric contraction by straightening out and propelling you upward. This conversion, let's say, takes exactly one second to complete. Your legs have to absorb the shock of going forward by bending, an eccentric contraction, then your legs have to overcome this force, and convert this exact same energy into half a second, instead of one second, then your force would be doubled. The half of a second that was saved would then be converted into height, or air time.

Let me explain quickly, three types of contractions that take place during this conversion cycle: eccentric, isometric, and concentric. An eccentric contraction takes place when the muscles undergo a force that is greater than the muscles are exerting. It, therefore, "gives" under this force and is stretched or lengthened. I like to remember this by saying it becomes "elastic" or "stretched." Thus, an eccentric (elastic) contraction is the lengthening of the muscles. An isometric contraction is next. The muscle is contracted, but there is no movement in any direction. Isometric contractions are "isolated," or not going anywhere. A concentric contraction is last and this occurs when the muscle generates more force than what is acting upon it, and it moves the weight in the opposite direction. In a concentric contraction, the muscle contracts, and becomes shorter.

A good example of an eccentric contraction would be the dropping of a tennis ball and a golf ball from the same height onto a concrete floor. The tension of the golf ball is harder, or stronger, than that of a tennis ball. The covering of the golf ball is compressed harder, therefore it doesn't "give" as much when it hits the floor. It therefore bounces higher. The stronger your eccentric contraction, the less stretching it will undergo and the higher you can jump, or the faster you can run.

FORCE = MASS ACCELERATION

F = 180 lbs. x 2A, A is now twice as fast

FORCE = 360 LBS.

2 times as fast = half (1/2) the time

2 times as fast = 8 minutes x 1/2 the time

2 times as fast = 4 minutes

Run Faster and Jump Higher, Naturally

Stretching and a low body fat ratio are the two most important factors that can contribute best toward running faster and jumping higher, naturally.

Stretching incorporates flexibility of the muscle groups by giving them full range of motion. Muscles are able to absorb energy quicker in the eccentric contraction through the entire length of the muscle, and release energy during the concentric contraction. Gymnasts, male and female, are very muscular, yet their flexibility and explosive power is fantastic.

A low body fat ratio is also critical. If a pro runner has a 6% body fat ratio, which means his total body weight consists of only 6% fat, imagine how much faster he could run if he was to lose five pounds of fat and yet keep his explosive strength. He would weigh less and therefore be able to propel his body forward faster.

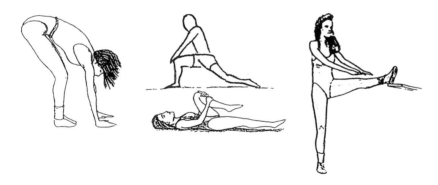

Always stretch first!

A 300-pound football player runs a 5.0-second 40-yard dash. If he was to lose twenty or thirty pounds of body fat and yet maintain his strength, he would be much more effective. He would be much faster and would probably be able to run a 4.6-second 40-yard dash. If he could do this, I'd make him a running back.

100% Exertion Needs 48 Hours
for 100% Recovery

I'm a firm believer that a high intensity, 100% effort workout is far better than a 90% effort workout, even when the 90% workout is repeated several times.

I can use the example of a runner and a swimmer. If I ran 200 meters in 20 seconds, which was 100% effort, and I was completely exhausted to the point where my legs had collapsed, or almost collapsed, this would be considered a high intensity workout. I personally don't want to train like this because of the pain, so I decided to run 200 meters at 90%, or let's say 25 seconds, but I'll do it three or four times so I can have a longer workout and, of course, experience less pain. Actually, it's better to run all out, 100% effort, than even twenty attempts at 90%! It doesn't matter how many times I run the 200 meters at 90%, or even 95%, because only a 100% effort forces muscles to overcompensate, to grow, and to get stronger.

I'm not sure how many hours world-class sprinters around the world train, but I do know that swimmers train for hours at a time, several times a day, and swim up to 10,000 meters a day or more. I know this because I did this for six years in junior high and high school. During all those hours of swimming lap after lap, I probably didn't exert more than 80% total effort at any one time, even though I had to repeat "timed" laps up to eight times. I do realize that if my coaches knew what I know now, I should have been swimming at 100%, which is what I did in every race, instead of swimming for hours and only building up endurance. The only way to prepare for 100%, is to train 100%!

Now, if only I wasn't so tired the next day, I'd be able to train just as hard every day, five days in a row. STOP! The reason I'm so tired is because my body hasn't recovered from this 100% exertion. If I was to run until failure, or swim until failure, my muscles would be able to recuperate up to 50% in about three seconds, but it would take around forty-eight hours to recuperate up to 100%. If I was to do another strenuous workout before I recovered, then my muscles wouldn't get the chance to grow, and they would never recover to 100% until I got that rest.

I'm a firm believer in a three-day-a-week training schedule. If you were to workout on Monday, Wednesday, and Friday, your body would become used to the routine of a workout every other day. Your body would then anticipate and gear up for the next workout, on Sunday, but you would not work out on Sunday. This throws your body into shock, keeping it from becoming used to a weekly routine and preventing you from falling into a rut.

There is a way to train five days a week or more. You must train every other day, three days a week, at 100%, and you would only stretch and work on "form," lightly, on the days in between.

Let's Learn the Exercises and Get Down to Business!

Preconditioning

I'd like to assume that you are already in good condition. If you are or are not in good shape, it is necessary that the following conditioning drills be accomplished before continuing. I suggest wind sprints between 30 and 50 yards, between five and ten repetitions (or more), with only thirty seconds of rest between sprints, done every other day for a week. A sprint called a "suicide sprint" can be done on a basketball court. Run from one line to another and back again, then run to another line farther away and back again. Run back and forth until three or more lines are touched up to five times at a 100% effort. Once this exercise is mastered and has been done correctly for one week, continue to the next exercises.

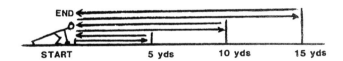

Suicide sprints

Height Jumping

Height jumping involves the eccentric contraction of the leg muscles by jumping from different heights. Jumping down from different heights incorporates different levels of maximum eccentric contractions. Each level generates maximum tension in the

37

legs and hips by generating forces that are up to twenty times greater than the athlete's own body weight. The higher the height, the greater the force exerted. I suggest landing on a mat of some kind or landing in sand to help prevent any shock to the soles of the feet, ankles, and knee ligaments. The exercise should be executed exactly as follows, even for world-class athletes. The athlete steps off from the following heights and lands with a minimum amount of bending in the knees, and without having the knees in a locked position. A bleacher is excellent for the various heights, and is found in gyms and at athletic fields all over America.

Light jogging over short distances should follow each set to keep the legs loose from the previous stress, and the sets should be done within one minute of each other. Any soreness in the feet, ankles, knees, or hips should be taken seriously. The exercise should be stopped, and anti-inflammatory measures should be taken.

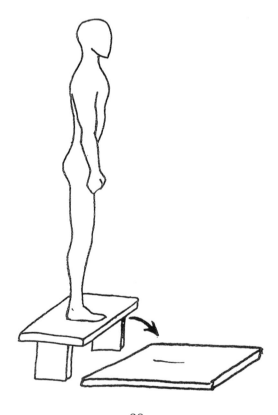

Week 1:

Monday—2-foot height   2 sets at 10 times each set
Wednesday—3-foot height   2 sets at 10 times each set
Friday—4-foot height   2 sets at 10 times each set

Week 2:

Monday—4-foot height   2 sets at 10 times each set
Wednesday—5-foot height   2 sets at 10 times each set
Friday—6-foot height   2 sets at 10 times each set

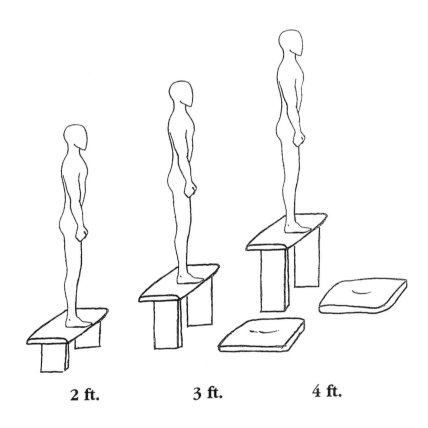

2 ft.   **3 ft.**   **4 ft.**

Height Jumping with Immediate Take-off

This exercise involves all three muscle contractions and should be done very carefully. The athlete steps off the bench, and with minimum bending in the knees, lands on both feet and immediately explodes upward by throwing the arms high over the head, reaching up as high as possible.

Light jogging should be done between each set with no more than one minute between each set. And once again, any soreness in the joints should be taken seriously!

No one should undergo any unnecessary stress or exercise on the days between the workout days. Basketball teams shouldn't do any strenuous running and jumping skills. Tennis, volleyball, baseball, football, and all other athletes should refrain from any strenuous running drills, to ensure proper rest.

Follow this exercise exactly as outlined.

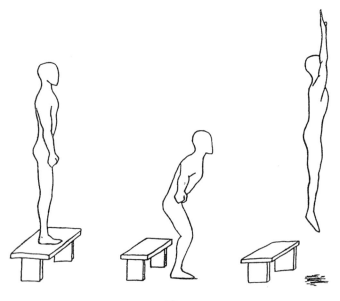

Week 1:

Monday—2-foot height   2 sets 10 times each set
Wednesday—2-foot height   2 sets 15 times each set
Friday—2-foot height   2 sets 20 times each set

Week 2:

Monday—3-foot height   2 sets 10 times each set
Wednesday—3-foot height   2 sets 15 times each set
Friday—3-foot height   2 sets 20 times each set

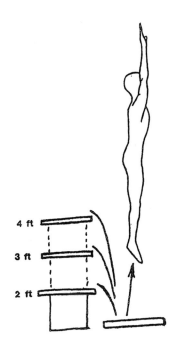

Hopping

Hopping incorporates all three contractions also, except now we are going to convert all forces into "forward" movement. Hopping is the closest you can get to actual running, and the forces exerted are far greater. Two-legged hops are performed first, and only when this exercise is mastered can the athlete then perform one-legged hops. Two-legged hops overload the leg muscles, and I consider this a preconditioning for the one-legged hops. One-legged hops overload the legs individually, creating even greater, but equal, development. Most people favor one leg or the other when performing a jump, therefore equal development enhances a double-leg jump.

I've seen, and performed some hopping exercises that incorporate jumping over chairs and boxes of different heights. This provides variety to the jumping exercises, but I prefer to hop over a measured distance for times, like wind sprints. The athlete should attempt to beat their previous fast time to ensure 100% effort when performing the following program.

Hopping drills over long distances can become an exhausting task and make you very clumsy. Tying your shoelaces together during the two-legged drills will help you keep your feet together.

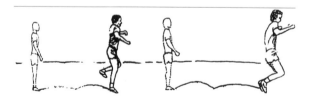

1- and 2-legged hops

42

Light jogging between each set, with no more than one minute between each set.

Week 1:

Monday—3 sets for time	Approx. 30 yards, using 2 legs
Wednesday—4 sets for time	Approx. 30 yards, using 2 legs
Friday—5 sets for time	Approx. 30 yards, using 2 legs

Week 2:

Monday—3 sets for time	Approx. 60 yards, using 2 legs
Wednesday—4 sets for time	Approx. 60 yards, using 2 legs
Friday—5 sets for time	Approx. 60 yards, using 2 legs

Week 3:

Monday—3 sets for time	Approx. 30 yards, using 1 leg for 3 sets, then the other leg.
Wednesday—4 sets for time	Approx. 30 yards, using 1 leg for 4 sets, then the other leg.
Friday—5 sets for time	Approx. 30 yards, using 1 leg for 5 sets, then the other leg.

Week 4:

Monday—3 sets for time	Approx. 60 yards, using 1 leg for 3 sets, then the other leg.
Wednesday—4 sets for time	Approx. 60 yards, using 1 leg for 4 sets, then the other leg.
Friday—5 sets for time	Approx. 60 yards, using 1 leg for 5 sets, then the other leg.

Running Downhill

Anyone can run downhill faster than they can run the same distance on a flat surface or uphill; this is common sense. Then why don't coaches have their athletes run down a hill as part of their training? I don't know! Maybe some coaches do make their teams run downhill, but I've never heard or seen it anywhere, and I've never read about it either.

I asked someone the other day the first thing he would do to make himself run faster if he was to start training. He said he would start running up hills and up long stairways. Ten out of ten people would probably say the same thing, but it's not so true. Running up stairs or running uphill shortens the leg muscles and this will actually make you run slower when on a flat surface. The benefits you will get from running up stairs or uphill are increased strength and endurance, but not explosive strength, which is necessary for sprinting and jumping.

The Chicago Bears had one of the greatest professional running backs ever. He had the most grueling uphill running training program that anyone would ever want to attempt. This uphill training gave him great strength and endurance, but he wasn't really known for his speed. If he had finished his workout by running downhill, and had increased his speed by even just a little, imagine what records he could have broken.

If you were able to find a steep hill or bridge to run down, the first thing you would notice is that running downhill causes you to lose your balance. You, in turn, must slow your pace and lean backward, so that you won't fall forward, flat on your face. It's hard to train for speed on a hill when you're doing somersaults, head first, so let's start near the bottom of the hill instead of the top. Measure two marks that are 40 yards apart; have this at only a slight incline. Do several sprints down the incline, hopefully without falling, and time them. You should be able to run

44

full speed without feeling yourself leaning backwards to keep balance. Your times will be faster than any previous 40-yard dash you have run; your legs are responding faster than ever before, your stride length is being increased naturally, and since muscles have memory, you will be able to run a 40-yard dash on a flat surface faster than before. But let's not stop there! Let's now increase the steepness by only 10 yards or so, depending on how steep your hill or bridge is, and again, not so steep that you could lose your balance or hold yourself back from a full sprint. By all means, don't limit yourself to 40-yard dashes. Feel free to run sprints of 100 yards or more, even 400 meters, if you can find a hill or bridge that would allow you to sprint at full speed without falling.

Actual Workout

I believe that athletes of all sports should precondition them-
selves before their season begins by completing all of the above
exercises in order. Once their season actually starts, their training can be adjusting to only hopping and running downhill.

Week 1: Preconditioning

Monday, Wednesday, Friday.
Run five sprints between 30-50 yards with thirty-second rests
between sprints, or run "suicides" five times or more. Run uphill
or run stadium stairs for endurance, strength, and not speed.

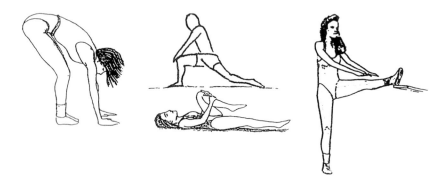

Always stretch first!

Week 2: Height Jumping

Monday—2-foot height   2 sets 10 times each
Wednesday—3-foot height   2 sets 10 times each
Friday—4-foot height   2 sets 10 times each

46

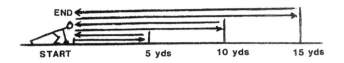

Suicide sprints

Week 3:

Monday—4-foot height   2 sets 10 times each
Wednesday—5-foot height   2 sets 10 times each
Friday—6-foot height   2 sets 10 times each

(Allow no more than fifteen seconds rest between each jump, and 1-2 minutes rest between each set.)

Here is a slower pace to follow for height jumping.

Week 2:

Monday—2-foot height   2 sets 10 times each
Wednesday—2-foot height   2 sets 15 times each
Friday—3-foot height   2 sets 10 times each

Week 3:

Monday—3-foot height   2 sets 15 times each
Wednesday—4-foot height   2 sets 10 times each
Friday—4-foot height   2 sets 15 times each

Week 4:

Monday—5-foot height   2 sets 10 times each
Wednesday—5-foot height   2 sets 15 times each
Friday—6-foot height   2 sets 10 times each

(Allow no more than fifteen seconds rest between each jump, and 1-2 minutes rest between each set.)

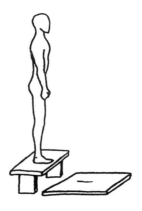

Week 4: Height Jumping with Take-off

Monday—2-foot height	2 sets 10 times each
Wednesday—2-foot height	2 sets 15 times each
Friday—2-foot height	2 sets 20 times each

Week 5:

Monday—3-foot height	2 sets 10 times each
Wednesday—3-foot height	2 sets 15 times each
Friday—3-foot height	2 sets 20 times each

(Allow no more than 15 seconds rest between each jump, and 1-2 minutes rest between each set.)

Week 6: Hopping

Monday—3 sets, 30 yards or more, 2-legged hops
Wednesday—4 sets, 30 yards or more, 2-legged hops
Friday—5 sets, 30 yards or more, 2-legged hops

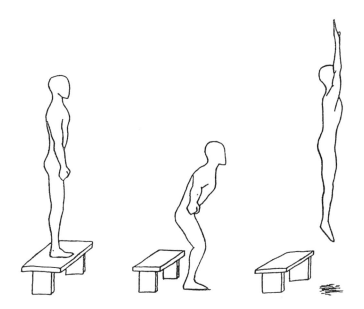

Week 7:

Monday—3 sets, 60 yards or more, 2-legged hops
Wednesday—4 sets, 60 yards or more, 2-legged hops
Friday—5 sets, 60 yards or more, 2-legged hops

Week 8:

Monday—3 sets, 30 yards or more, 1-legged hops
Wednesday—4 sets, 30 yards or more, 1-legged hops
Friday—5 sets, 30 yards or more, 1-legged hops

Week 9:

Monday—3 sets, 60 yards or more, 1-legged hops
Wednesday—4 sets, 60 yards or more, 1-legged hops
Friday—5 sets, 60 yards or more, 1-legged hops

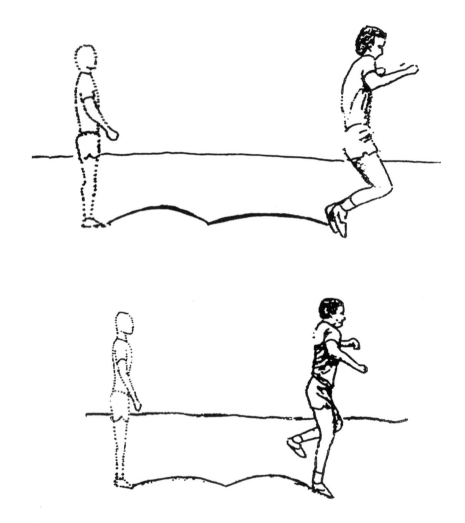

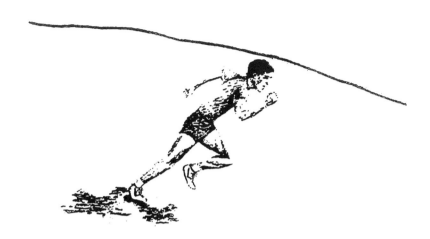

(A 30-second rest between each set, or the hops can be alternated from one leg to the other without rest until three sets on each is completed. Each set should be timed to ensure full speed.)

Week 10:

Downhill sprints can be done following this pre-season workout. It can be done "during" the season and year round. Individuals can create their own downhill training, as long as the sprinting is at full speed.

All sports use some kind of explosive power, whether it occurs in the legs and/or upper body. Each sport requires specific training and specific plyometric exercises, but actual test results are not available at this time. General guidelines for some sports are as follows, and coaches are more than welcome to develop their own training schedules based on their trial-and-error data.

Sprinters should use the previous training outline for their pre-season workout. Their in-season training should incorporate two-legged hopping, then one-legged (timing speeds at various distances, from 20 up to 400 meters, depending on the length of your sprint event). Downhill running should also be done where hills and bridges are available.

Football and baseball players should also follow the

pre-season schedule, and their in-season workout should consist of two-legged, then one-legged, hops. Football players can hop anywhere between 30 yards to 100 yards. Linemen should stay within 50 yards. Baseball players can do hopping sprints, two-legged then one-legged, from one base to another for faster times.

Volleyball and basketball players should use this pre-season workout and use "Height Jumping with Take-off" during their season. A two-legged, and then a one-legged, hopping workout should also be done during their in-season training.

Tennis players should complete their pre-season workout and use two-legged, and then one-legged, hops during their season.

Swimmers and wrestlers can use the pre-season workout, but I wouldn't consider it necessary. A two-legged, and then one-legged, hopping workout should be followed, however, throughout the entire season.

Snow skiers and speed skaters should do extremely strenuous hopping exercises. Two-legged, and then one-legged, hops should be performed, gradually building up to 400 meters or more.

All athletes, including long-distance runners, must run downhill as far as the distance of their event, as fast as possible. Mile runners should run one-mile sprints downhill, 400-meter runners should run sprints down a 400-meter hill, etc. Marathon runners should train in the mountains, running downhill (never uphill) as far as possible, up to 26 miles. If there is a downhill stretch 26 miles long somewhere in America, I can guarantee that soon you won't be the only one running down that hill.

If weight training is an integral part of your sports conditioning, it must be done last. All explosive exercises must be done first, when you are at your strongest, then downhill sprints and then weight training, always in this order only—on the same day—every other day!